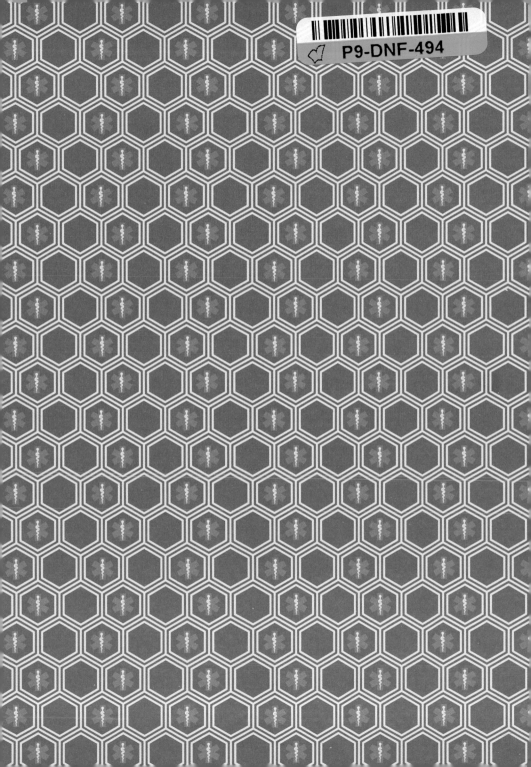

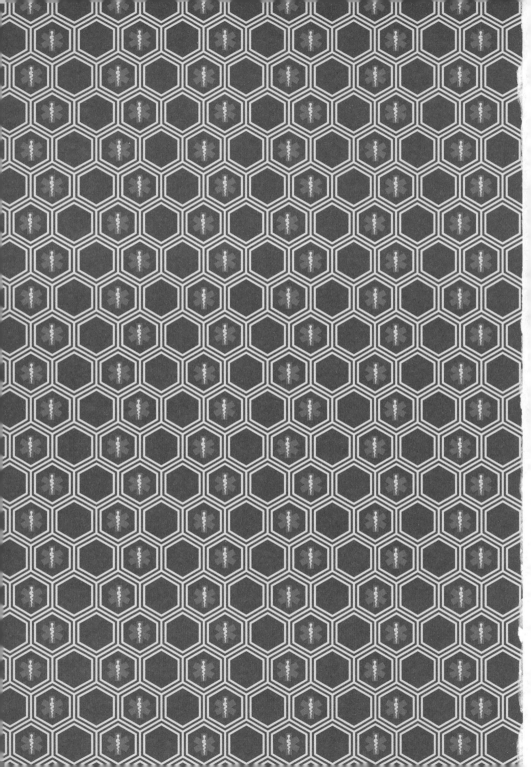

My Personal Health Record Keeper

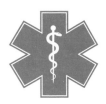

PETER PAUPER PRESS, INC.
WHITE PLAINS, NEW YORK

PETER PAUPER PRESS
Fine Books and Gifts Since 1928

Our Company

In 1928, at the age of twenty-two, Peter Beilenson began printing books on a small press in the basement of his parents' home in Larchmont, New York. Peter—and later, his wife, Edna—sought to create fine books that sold at "prices even a pauper could afford."

Today, still family owned and operated, Peter Pauper Press continues to honor our founders' legacy—and our customers' expectations—of beauty, quality, and value.

Designed by Tesslyn Pandarakalam
Images used under license from Shutterstock.com

Visit us at www.peterpauper.com

The publisher has made every effort to ensure the accuracy of the information in this health record keeper. Nonetheless, medical information changes frequently, and we advise the reader to consult a physician in matters relating to health. Peter Pauper Press cannot be held liable for any errors, omissions, or inconsistencies.

CONTENTS

My Profile Snapshot

Name:

Date of Birth: .... Blood Type: ....

Height: .... Weight: ....

ASSISTIVE DEVICES:

....

....

MEDICAL CONDITIONS:

....

....

....

....

ALLERGIES:

Medication	Reaction

EMERGENCY CONTACT:

Name: ....

Phone: ....

Alternate Phone: ....

Relationship: ....

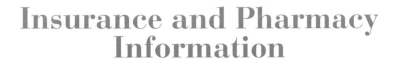

Insurance and Pharmacy Information

Insurance Company Name:

Insurance Plan Name:

Group #:

ID #:

Member Services Phone #:

Insurance Company Name:

Insurance Plan Name:

Group #:

ID #:

Member Services Phone #:

Current Pharmacy:

Phone:

Fax:

Address:

Alternate Pharmacy:

Phone:

Fax:

Address:

Doctors' & Specialists' Information

PRIMARY CARE PHYSICIAN

Name:

Phone:

Address:

OB-GYN

Name:

Phone:

Address:

DENTIST

Name:

Phone:

Address:

EYE DOCTOR

Name:

Phone:

Address:

SPECIALIST (_____)

Name:

Phone:

Address:

SPECIALIST (_____)

Name:

Phone:

Address:

SPECIALIST (_____)

Name:

Phone:

Address:

SPECIALIST (_____)

Name:

Phone:

Address:

Family Health History

MOTHER'S FAMILY: GENETIC OR MEDICAL CONDITIONS

Name	Relation	Condition & date of onset

FATHER'S FAMILY: GENETIC OR MEDICAL CONDITIONS

Name	Relation	Condition & date of onset

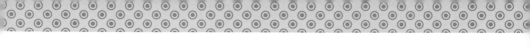

SIBLING(S): GENETIC OR MEDICAL CONDITIONS

Name	Relation	Condition & date of onset

Surgery, Hospitalization, & Emergency Room Records

SURGERIES:

Type	Surgeon	Date

HOSPITALIZATIONS:

Reason	Hospital	Date

EMERGENCY ROOM VISITS:

Reason	Facility	Date

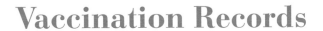

Vaccination Records

Vaccination requirements may vary. Please check with your doctor.

Vaccine	Recommended	Date	Date	Date	Date
Td Booster	Every 10 yrs				
Tdap	1 Dose				
Varicella	2 Doses				
Meningococccal	1 Dose				
MMR	1 or 2 Doses				
Hepatitis A	2 Doses				
Hepatitis B	3 Doses				
HPV	3 Doses				
Shingles	1 Dose				
Pneumonia	1 or 2 Doses				
Flu	Yearly				

Medications, Vitamins, & Supplements

Name:

Dosage: Frequency:

Date started: Date ended:

Side effects:

Name:

Dosage: Frequency:

Date started: Date ended:

Side effects:

Name:

Dosage: Frequency:

Date started: Date ended:

Side effects:

Name:

Dosage: Frequency:

Date started: Date ended:

Side effects:

Name:

Dosage: Frequency:

Date started: Date ended:

Side effects:

Name:

Dosage: Frequency:

Date started: Date ended:

Side effects:

Name:

Dosage: Frequency:

Date started: Date ended:

Side effects:

Name:

Dosage: Frequency:

Date started: Date ended:

Side effects:

Name:

Dosage: Frequency:

Date started: Date ended:

Side effects:

Name:

Dosage: Frequency:

Date started: Date ended:

Side effects:

Medications, Vitamins, & Supplements

Name:

Dosage: Frequency:

Date started: Date ended:

Side effects:

Name:

Dosage: Frequency:

Date started: Date ended:

Side effects:

Name:

Dosage: Frequency:

Date started: Date ended:

Side effects:

Name:

Dosage: Frequency:

Date started: Date ended:

Side effects:

Name:

Dosage: Frequency:

Date started: Date ended:

Side effects:

Name:

Dosage: Frequency:

Date started: Date ended:

Side effects:

Name:

Dosage: Frequency:

Date started: Date ended:

Side effects:

Name:

Dosage: Frequency:

Date started: Date ended:

Side effects:

Name:

Dosage: Frequency:

Date started: Date ended:

Side effects:

Name:

Dosage: Frequency:

Date started: Date ended:

Side effects:

Medications, Vitamins, & Supplements

Name:

Dosage: Frequency:

Date started: Date ended:

Side effects:

Name:

Dosage: Frequency:

Date started: Date ended:

Side effects:

Name:

Dosage: Frequency:

Date started: Date ended:

Side effects:

Name:

Dosage: Frequency:

Date started: Date ended:

Side effects:

Name:

Dosage: Frequency:

Date started: Date ended:

Side effects:

Name:

Dosage: Frequency:

Date started: Date ended:

Side effects:

Name:

Dosage: Frequency:

Date started: Date ended:

Side effects:

Name:

Dosage: Frequency:

Date started: Date ended:

Side effects:

Name:

Dosage: Frequency:

Date started: Date ended:

Side effects:

Name:

Dosage: Frequency:

Date started: Date ended:

Side effects:

Vision History

VISUAL ACUITY:

Left Eye: _____ Right Eye: _____ Date: _____

Left Eye: _____ Right Eye: _____ Date: _____

Left Eye: _____ Right Eye: _____ Date: _____

Left Eye: _____ Right Eye: _____ Date: _____

Left Eye: _____ Right Eye: _____ Date: _____

Left Eye: _____ Right Eye: _____ Date: _____

Left Eye: _____ Right Eye: _____ Date: _____

Left Eye: _____ Right Eye: _____ Date: _____

NOTES

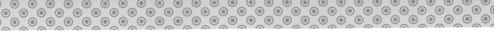

Dental History

List types and dates of dental surgeries, procedures, and any other relevant dental information.

Description of ailment:

Date of onset and duration:

Treatment:

What were you doing at the onset?

Description of ailment:

Date of onset and duration:

Treatment:

What were you doing at the onset?

Description of ailment:

Date of onset and duration:

Treatment:

What were you doing at the onset?

Description of ailment:

Date of onset and duration:

Treatment:

What were you doing at the onset?

Description of ailment:

Date of onset and duration:

Treatment:

What were you doing at the onset?

Description of ailment:

Date of onset and duration:

Treatment:

What were you doing at the onset?

Description of ailment:

Date of onset and duration:

Treatment:

What were you doing at the onset?

Description of ailment:

Date of onset and duration:

Treatment:

What were you doing at the onset?

Description of ailment:

Date of onset and duration:

Treatment:

What were you doing at the onset?

Description of ailment:

Date of onset and duration:

Treatment:

What were you doing at the onset?

Description of ailment:

Date of onset and duration:

Treatment:

What were you doing at the onset?

Description of ailment:

Date of onset and duration:

Treatment:

What were you doing at the onset?

Description of ailment:

Date of onset and duration:

Treatment:

What were you doing at the onset?

Description of ailment:

Date of onset and duration:

Treatment:

What were you doing at the onset?

Description of ailment:

Date of onset and duration:

Treatment:

What were you doing at the onset?

Description of ailment:

Date of onset and duration:

Treatment:

What were you doing at the onset?

Description of ailment:

Date of onset and duration:

Treatment:

What were you doing at the onset?

Description of ailment:

Date of onset and duration:

Treatment:

What were you doing at the onset?

Description of ailment:

Date of onset and duration:

Treatment:

What were you doing at the onset?

Description of ailment:

Date of onset and duration:

Treatment:

What were you doing at the onset?

Description of ailment:

Date of onset and duration:

Treatment:

What were you doing at the onset?

Description of ailment:

Date of onset and duration:

Treatment:

What were you doing at the onset?

Description of ailment:

Date of onset and duration:

Treatment:

What were you doing at the onset?

Description of ailment:

Date of onset and duration:

Treatment:

What were you doing at the onset?

Description of ailment:

Date of onset and duration:

Treatment:

What were you doing at the onset?

Description of ailment:

Date of onset and duration:

Treatment:

What were you doing at the onset?

Description of ailment:

Date of onset and duration:

Treatment:

What were you doing at the onset?

Description of ailment:

Date of onset and duration:

Treatment:

What were you doing at the onset?

Description of ailment:

Date of onset and duration:

Treatment:

What were you doing at the onset?

Description of ailment:

Date of onset and duration:

Treatment:

What were you doing at the onset?

Description of ailment:

Date of onset and duration:

Treatment:

What were you doing at the onset?

Description of ailment:

Date of onset and duration:

Treatment:

What were you doing at the onset?

Description of ailment:

Date of onset and duration:

Treatment:

What were you doing at the onset?

Description of ailment:

Date of onset and duration:

Treatment:

What were you doing at the onset?

Description of ailment:

Date of onset and duration:

Treatment:

What were you doing at the onset?

Description of ailment:

Date of onset and duration:

Treatment:

What were you doing at the onset?

Description of ailment:

Date of onset and duration:

Treatment:

What were you doing at the onset?

Description of ailment:

Date of onset and duration:

Treatment:

What were you doing at the onset?

Description of ailment:

Date of onset and duration:

Treatment:

What were you doing at the onset?

Description of ailment:

Date of onset and duration:

Treatment:

What were you doing at the onset?

Description of ailment:

Date of onset and duration:

Treatment:

What were you doing at the onset?

Description of ailment:

Date of onset and duration:

Treatment:

What were you doing at the onset?

Description of ailment:

Date of onset and duration:

Treatment:

What were you doing at the onset?

Description of ailment:

Date of onset and duration:

Treatment:

What were you doing at the onset?

Description of ailment:

Date of onset and duration:

Treatment:

What were you doing at the onset?

Description of ailment:

Date of onset and duration:

Treatment:

What were you doing at the onset?

Description of ailment:

Date of onset and duration:

Treatment:

What were you doing at the onset?

Description of ailment:

Date of onset and duration:

Treatment:

What were you doing at the onset?

Description of ailment:

Date of onset and duration:

Treatment:

What were you doing at the onset?

Description of ailment:

Date of onset and duration:

Treatment:

What were you doing at the onset?

Description of ailment:

Date of onset and duration:

Treatment:

What were you doing at the onset?

Description of ailment:

Date of onset and duration:

Treatment:

What were you doing at the onset?

Description of ailment:

Date of onset and duration:

Treatment:

What were you doing at the onset?

Description of ailment:

Date of onset and duration:

Treatment:

What were you doing at the onset?

Description of ailment:

Date of onset and duration:

Treatment:

What were you doing at the onset?

Description of ailment:

Date of onset and duration:

Treatment:

What were you doing at the onset?

Description of ailment:

Date of onset and duration:

Treatment:

What were you doing at the onset?

Ailments History

Description of ailment:

Date of onset and duration:

Treatment:

What were you doing at the onset?

Description of ailment:

Date of onset and duration:

Treatment:

What were you doing at the onset?

Description of ailment:

Date of onset and duration:

Treatment:

What were you doing at the onset?

Description of ailment:

Date of onset and duration:

Treatment:

What were you doing at the onset?

Description of ailment:

Date of onset and duration:

Treatment:

What were you doing at the onset?

Description of ailment:

Date of onset and duration:

Treatment:

What were you doing at the onset?

Description of ailment:

Date of onset and duration:

Treatment:

What were you doing at the onset?

Description of ailment:

Date of onset and duration:

Treatment:

What were you doing at the onset?

Description of ailment:

Date of onset and duration:

Treatment:

What were you doing at the onset?

Description of ailment:

Date of onset and duration:

Treatment:

What were you doing at the onset?

Description of ailment:

Date of onset and duration:

Treatment:

What were you doing at the onset?

Description of ailment:

Date of onset and duration:

Treatment:

What were you doing at the onset?

Description of ailment:

Date of onset and duration:

Treatment:

What were you doing at the onset?

Description of ailment:

Date of onset and duration:

Treatment:

What were you doing at the onset?

Description of ailment:

Date of onset and duration:

Treatment:

What were you doing at the onset?

Description of ailment:

Date of onset and duration:

Treatment:

What were you doing at the onset?

Description of ailment:

Date of onset and duration:

Treatment:

What were you doing at the onset?

Description of ailment:

Date of onset and duration:

Treatment:

What were you doing at the onset?

Description of ailment:

Date of onset and duration:

Treatment:

What were you doing at the onset?

Description of ailment:

Date of onset and duration:

Treatment:

What were you doing at the onset?

Description of ailment:

Date of onset and duration:

Treatment:

What were you doing at the onset?

OFFICE VISIT

Date: .... Doctor: ....

Phone: .... Address: ....

Reason for visit: ....

....

....

....

Doctor's diagnosis/feedback: ....

....

....

....

Test ordered: .... Test result: ....

....

....

....

....

Weight: .... Blood pressure: ....

Temperature: .... Heart rate: ....

Prescribed treatment:

Prescribed medications, vitamins, supplements:

Name: Dosage:

Frequency: Duration:

With meal and/or water?

Possible side effects:

NOTES

OFFICE VISIT

Date: Doctor:

Phone: Address:

Reason for visit:

Doctor's diagnosis/feedback:

Test ordered: Test result:

Weight: Blood pressure:

Temperature: Heart rate:

Prescribed treatment:

Prescribed medications, vitamins, supplements:

Name: Dosage:

Frequency: Duration:

With meal and/or water?

Possible side effects:

NOTES

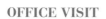

OFFICE VISIT

Date: _____ Doctor: _____

Phone: _____ Address: _____

_____

Reason for visit: _____

_____

_____

_____

_____

Doctor's diagnosis/feedback: _____

_____

_____

_____

_____

_____

Test ordered: Test result:

_____   _____

_____   _____

_____   _____

_____   _____

_____   _____

Weight: _____ Blood pressure: _____

Temperature: _____ Heart rate: _____

Prescribed treatment:

Prescribed medications, vitamins, supplements:

Name: Dosage:

Frequency: Duration:

With meal and/or water?

Possible side effects:

NOTES

OFFICE VISIT

Date: _____   Doctor: _____

Phone: _____   Address: _____

Reason for visit:
_____
_____
_____
_____

Doctor's diagnosis/feedback:
_____
_____
_____
_____

Test ordered: Test result:
_____   _____
_____   _____
_____   _____
_____   _____

Weight: _____   Blood pressure: _____

Temperature: _____   Heart rate: _____

Prescribed treatment:

Prescribed medications, vitamins, supplements:

Name: Dosage:

Frequency: Duration:

With meal and/or water?

Possible side effects:

NOTES

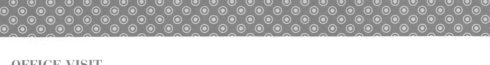

OFFICE VISIT

Date: Doctor:

Phone: Address:

Reason for visit:

Doctor's diagnosis/feedback:

Test ordered: Test result:

Weight: Blood pressure:

Temperature: Heart rate:

Prescribed treatment:

....

....

....

....

....

Prescribed medications, vitamins, supplements:

Name: Dosage:

Frequency: Duration:

With meal and/or water?

Possible side effects:

....

NOTES

OFFICE VISIT

Date: Doctor:

Phone: Address:

Reason for visit:

Doctor's diagnosis/feedback:

Test ordered: Test result:

Weight: Blood pressure:

Temperature: Heart rate:

Prescribed treatment:

Prescribed medications, vitamins, supplements:

Name: Dosage:

Frequency: Duration:

With meal and/or water?

Possible side effects:

NOTES

OFFICE VISIT

Date: Doctor:

Phone: Address:

Reason for visit:

Doctor's diagnosis/feedback:

Test ordered: Test result:

Weight: Blood pressure:

Temperature: Heart rate:

Prescribed treatment:

Prescribed medications, vitamins, supplements:

Name: Dosage:

Frequency: Duration:

With meal and/or water?

Possible side effects:

NOTES

OFFICE VISIT

Date: Doctor:

Phone: Address:

Reason for visit:

Doctor's diagnosis/feedback:

Test ordered: Test result:

Weight: Blood pressure:

Temperature: Heart rate:

Prescribed treatment:

Prescribed medications, vitamins, supplements:

Name: Dosage:

Frequency: Duration:

With meal and/or water?

Possible side effects:

NOTES

OFFICE VISIT

Date: Doctor:

Phone: Address:

Reason for visit:

Doctor's diagnosis/feedback:

Test ordered: Test result:

Weight: Blood pressure:

Temperature: Heart rate:

Prescribed treatment:

Prescribed medications, vitamins, supplements:

Name: Dosage:

Frequency: Duration:

With meal and/or water?

Possible side effects:

NOTES

OFFICE VISIT

Date: .... Doctor: ....

Phone: .... Address: ....

....

Reason for visit:

....

....

....

....

Doctor's diagnosis/feedback:

....

....

....

....

Test ordered: Test result:

....

....

....

....

Weight: .... Blood pressure: ....

Temperature: .... Heart rate: ....

Prescribed treatment:

Prescribed medications, vitamins, supplements:

Name: Dosage:

Frequency: Duration:

With meal and/or water?

Possible side effects:

NOTES

OFFICE VISIT

Date: Doctor:

Phone: Address:

Reason for visit:

Doctor's diagnosis/feedback:

Test ordered: Test result:

Weight: Blood pressure:

Temperature: Heart rate:

Prescribed treatment:

Prescribed medications, vitamins, supplements:

Name: Dosage:

Frequency: Duration:

With meal and/or water?

Possible side effects:

NOTES

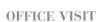

OFFICE VISIT

Date: .... Doctor: ....

Phone: .... Address: ....

....

Reason for visit: ....

....

....

....

....

Doctor's diagnosis/feedback: ....

....

....

....

....

....

Test ordered: .... Test result: ....

....

....

....

....

Weight: .... Blood pressure: ....

Temperature: .... Heart rate: ....

Prescribed treatment:

Prescribed medications, vitamins, supplements:

Name: Dosage:

Frequency: Duration:

With meal and/or water?

Possible side effects:

NOTES

OFFICE VISIT

Date: .... Doctor: ....

Phone: .... Address: ....

....

Reason for visit: ....

....

....

....

....

Doctor's diagnosis/feedback: ....

....

....

....

....

....

Test ordered: .... Test result: ....

....

....

....

....

Weight: .... Blood pressure: ....

Temperature: .... Heart rate: ....

Prescribed treatment:

Prescribed medications, vitamins, supplements:

Name: Dosage:

Frequency: Duration:

With meal and/or water?

Possible side effects:

NOTES

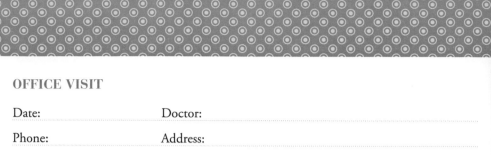

OFFICE VISIT

Date: Doctor:

Phone: Address:

Reason for visit:

Doctor's diagnosis/feedback:

Test ordered: Test result:

Weight: Blood pressure:

Temperature: Heart rate:

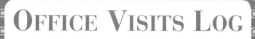

Prescribed treatment:

Prescribed medications, vitamins, supplements:

Name: Dosage:

Frequency: Duration:

With meal and/or water?

Possible side effects:

NOTES

OFFICE VISIT

Date: Doctor:

Phone: Address:

Reason for visit:

Doctor's diagnosis/feedback:

Test ordered: Test result:

Weight: Blood pressure:

Temperature: Heart rate:

Prescribed treatment:

Prescribed medications, vitamins, supplements:

Name: Dosage:

Frequency: Duration:

With meal and/or water?

Possible side effects:

NOTES

OFFICE VISIT

Date: .... Doctor: ....

Phone: .... Address: ....

....

Reason for visit: ....

....

....

....

....

Doctor's diagnosis/feedback: ....

....

....

....

....

Test ordered: .... Test result: ....

....

....

....

....

Weight: .... Blood pressure: ....

Temperature: .... Heart rate: ....

Prescribed treatment:

Prescribed medications, vitamins, supplements:

Name: Dosage:

Frequency: Duration:

With meal and/or water?

Possible side effects:

NOTES

OFFICE VISIT

Date: .... Doctor: ....

Phone: .... Address: ....

Reason for visit: ....

....

....

....

....

Doctor's diagnosis/feedback: ....

....

....

....

....

Test ordered: .... Test result: ....

....

....

....

....

Weight: .... Blood pressure: ....

Temperature: .... Heart rate: ....

Prescribed treatment:

Prescribed medications, vitamins, supplements:

Name: Dosage:

Frequency: Duration:

With meal and/or water?

Possible side effects:

NOTES

OFFICE VISIT

Date: .... Doctor: ....

Phone: .... Address: ....

Reason for visit: ....

....

....

....

Doctor's diagnosis/feedback: ....

....

....

....

....

Test ordered: .... Test result: ....

....

....

....

....

Weight: .... Blood pressure: ....

Temperature: .... Heart rate: ....

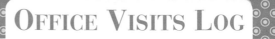

Prescribed treatment:

....

....

....

....

....

Prescribed medications, vitamins, supplements:

Name: .... Dosage: ....

Frequency: .... Duration: ....

With meal and/or water? ....

Possible side effects: ....

....

NOTES

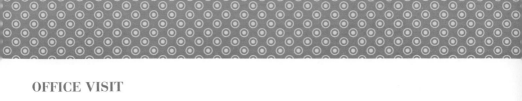

OFFICE VISIT

Date: .... Doctor: ....

Phone: .... Address: ....

....

Reason for visit: ....

....

....

....

....

Doctor's diagnosis/feedback: ....

....

....

....

....

Test ordered: .... Test result: ....

....

....

....

....

Weight: .... Blood pressure: ....

Temperature: .... Heart rate: ....

Prescribed treatment:

Prescribed medications, vitamins, supplements:

Name: Dosage:

Frequency: Duration:

With meal and/or water?

Possible side effects:

NOTES

OFFICE VISIT

Date: .... Doctor: ....

Phone: .... Address: ....

Reason for visit: ....

....

....

....

Doctor's diagnosis/feedback: ....

....

....

....

....

Test ordered: .... Test result: ....

....

....

....

....

Weight: .... Blood pressure: ....

Temperature: .... Heart rate: ....

Prescribed treatment:

Prescribed medications, vitamins, supplements:

Name: Dosage:

Frequency: Duration:

With meal and/or water?

Possible side effects:

NOTES

OFFICE VISIT

Date: .... Doctor: ....

Phone: .... Address: ....

Reason for visit: ....

....

....

....

....

Doctor's diagnosis/feedback: ....

....

....

....

....

....

Test ordered: .... Test result: ....

....

....

....

....

Weight: .... Blood pressure: ....

Temperature: .... Heart rate: ....

Prescribed treatment:

Prescribed medications, vitamins, supplements:

Name: Dosage:

Frequency: Duration:

With meal and/or water?

Possible side effects:

NOTES

OFFICE VISIT

Date: .... Doctor: ....

Phone: .... Address: ....

Reason for visit: ....

....

....

....

....

Doctor's diagnosis/feedback: ....

....

....

....

....

Test ordered: .... Test result: ....

....

....

....

....

Weight: .... Blood pressure: ....

Temperature: .... Heart rate: ....

Prescribed treatment:

Prescribed medications, vitamins, supplements:

Name: Dosage:

Frequency: Duration:

With meal and/or water?

Possible side effects:

NOTES

OFFICE VISIT

Date: .... Doctor: ....

Phone: .... Address: ....

Reason for visit: ....

....

....

....

Doctor's diagnosis/feedback: ....

....

....

....

....

Test ordered: .... Test result: ....

....

....

....

....

Weight: .... Blood pressure: ....

Temperature: .... Heart rate: ....

Prescribed treatment:

Prescribed medications, vitamins, supplements:

Name: Dosage:

Frequency: Duration:

With meal and/or water?

Possible side effects:

NOTES

OFFICE VISIT

Date: .... Doctor: ....

Phone: .... Address: ....

Reason for visit: ....

....

....

....

Doctor's diagnosis/feedback: ....

....

....

....

....

Test ordered: .... Test result: ....

....

....

....

....

Weight: .... Blood pressure: ....

Temperature: .... Heart rate: ....

Prescribed treatment:

Prescribed medications, vitamins, supplements:

Name: Dosage:

Frequency: Duration:

With meal and/or water?

Possible side effects:

NOTES

OFFICE VISIT

Date: _____ Doctor: _____

Phone: _____ Address: _____

_____

Reason for visit:

_____

_____

_____

_____

Doctor's diagnosis/feedback:

_____

_____

_____

_____

Test ordered: Test result:

_____   _____

_____   _____

_____   _____

_____   _____

Weight: _____ Blood pressure: _____

Temperature: _____ Heart rate: _____

Prescribed treatment:

Prescribed medications, vitamins, supplements:

Name: Dosage:

Frequency: Duration:

With meal and/or water?

Possible side effects:

NOTES

OFFICE VISIT

Date: .... Doctor: ....

Phone: .... Address: ....

....

Reason for visit: ....

....

....

....

....

Doctor's diagnosis/feedback: ....

....

....

....

....

Test ordered: .... Test result: ....

....

....

....

....

Weight: .... Blood pressure: ....

Temperature: .... Heart rate: ....

Prescribed treatment:

Prescribed medications, vitamins, supplements:

Name: Dosage:

Frequency: Duration:

With meal and/or water?

Possible side effects:

NOTES

OFFICE VISIT

Date: .... Doctor: ....

Phone: .... Address: ....

....

Reason for visit: ....

....

....

....

....

Doctor's diagnosis/feedback: ....

....

....

....

....

Test ordered: .... Test result: ....

....

....

....

....

Weight: .... Blood pressure: ....

Temperature: .... Heart rate: ....

Prescribed treatment:

Prescribed medications, vitamins, supplements:

Name: Dosage:

Frequency: Duration:

With meal and/or water?

Possible side effects:

NOTES

OFFICE VISIT

Date: .... Doctor: ....

Phone: .... Address: ....

....

Reason for visit: ....

....

....

....

....

Doctor's diagnosis/feedback: ....

....

....

....

....

Test ordered: .... Test result: ....

....

....

....

....

Weight: .... Blood pressure: ....

Temperature: .... Heart rate: ....

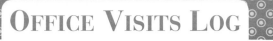

OFFICE VISITS LOG

Prescribed treatment:

Prescribed medications, vitamins, supplements:

Name: Dosage:

Frequency: Duration:

With meal and/or water?

Possible side effects:

NOTES

OFFICE VISIT

Date: Doctor:

Phone: Address:

Reason for visit:

Doctor's diagnosis/feedback:

Test ordered: Test result:

Weight: Blood pressure:

Temperature: Heart rate:

Prescribed treatment:

....

....

....

....

Prescribed medications, vitamins, supplements:

Name: Dosage:

Frequency: Duration:

With meal and/or water?

Possible side effects:

....

NOTES

OFFICE VISIT

Date: Doctor:

Phone: Address:

Reason for visit:

Doctor's diagnosis/feedback:

Test ordered: Test result:

Weight: Blood pressure:

Temperature: Heart rate:

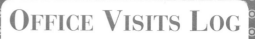

Prescribed treatment:

Prescribed medications, vitamins, supplements:

Name: Dosage:

Frequency: Duration:

With meal and/or water?

Possible side effects:

NOTES

OFFICE VISIT

Date: .... Doctor: ....

Phone: .... Address: ....

....

Reason for visit: ....

....

....

....

....

Doctor's diagnosis/feedback: ....

....

....

....

....

Test ordered: Test result:

....

....

....

....

....

Weight: .... Blood pressure: ....

Temperature: .... Heart rate: ....

Prescribed treatment:

Prescribed medications, vitamins, supplements:

Name: Dosage:

Frequency: Duration:

With meal and/or water?

Possible side effects:

NOTES

OFFICE VISIT

Date: .... Doctor: ....

Phone: .... Address: ....

Reason for visit: ....

....

....

....

Doctor's diagnosis/feedback: ....

....

....

....

Test ordered: .... Test result: ....

....

....

....

Weight: .... Blood pressure: ....

Temperature: .... Heart rate: ....

Prescribed treatment:

Prescribed medications, vitamins, supplements:

Name: Dosage:

Frequency: Duration:

With meal and/or water?

Possible side effects:

NOTES

OFFICE VISIT

Date: Doctor:

Phone: Address:

Reason for visit:

Doctor's diagnosis/feedback:

Test ordered: Test result:

Weight: Blood pressure:

Temperature: Heart rate:

Prescribed treatment:

Prescribed medications, vitamins, supplements:

Name: Dosage:

Frequency: Duration:

With meal and/or water?

Possible side effects:

NOTES

OFFICE VISIT

Date: Doctor:

Phone: Address:

Reason for visit:

Doctor's diagnosis/feedback:

Test ordered: Test result:

Weight: Blood pressure:

Temperature: Heart rate:

Prescribed treatment:

Prescribed medications, vitamins, supplements:

Name: Dosage:

Frequency: Duration:

With meal and/or water?

Possible side effects:

NOTES

OFFICE VISIT

Date: .... Doctor: ....

Phone: .... Address: ....

Reason for visit: ....

....

....

....

....

Doctor's diagnosis/feedback: ....

....

....

....

....

Test ordered: .... Test result: ....

....

....

....

....

Weight: .... Blood pressure: ....

Temperature: .... Heart rate: ....

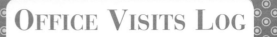
Prescribed treatment:

Prescribed medications, vitamins, supplements:

Name: Dosage:

Frequency: Duration:

With meal and/or water?

Possible side effects:

NOTES

OFFICE VISIT

Date: .... Doctor: ....

Phone: .... Address: ....

....

Reason for visit: ....

....

....

....

....

Doctor's diagnosis/feedback: ....

....

....

....

....

Test ordered: .... Test result: ....

....

....

....

....

Weight: .... Blood pressure: ....

Temperature: .... Heart rate: ....

Prescribed treatment:

Prescribed medications, vitamins, supplements:

Name: Dosage:

Frequency: Duration:

With meal and/or water?

Possible side effects:

NOTES

OFFICE VISIT

Date: Doctor:

Phone: Address:

Reason for visit:

Doctor's diagnosis/feedback:

Test ordered: Test result:

Weight: Blood pressure:

Temperature: Heart rate:

Prescribed treatment:

Prescribed medications, vitamins, supplements:

Name: Dosage:

Frequency: Duration:

With meal and/or water?

Possible side effects:

NOTES

OFFICE VISIT

Date: .... Doctor: ....

Phone: .... Address: ....

Reason for visit: ....

....

....

....

Doctor's diagnosis/feedback: ....

....

....

....

....

Test ordered: .... Test result: ....

....

....

....

....

Weight: .... Blood pressure: ....

Temperature: .... Heart rate: ....

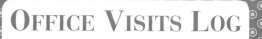
Prescribed treatment:

Prescribed medications, vitamins, supplements:

Name: Dosage:

Frequency: Duration:

With meal and/or water?

Possible side effects:

NOTES

OFFICE VISIT

Date: .... Doctor: ....

Phone: .... Address: ....

Reason for visit: ....

....

....

....

....

Doctor's diagnosis/feedback: ....

....

....

....

....

....

Test ordered: .... Test result: ....

....

....

....

....

....

Weight: .... Blood pressure: ....

Temperature: .... Heart rate: ....

Prescribed treatment:

Prescribed medications, vitamins, supplements:

Name: Dosage:

Frequency: Duration:

With meal and/or water?

Possible side effects:

NOTES

OFFICE VISIT

Date: .... Doctor: ....

Phone: .... Address: ....

Reason for visit: ....

....

....

....

Doctor's diagnosis/feedback: ....

....

....

....

Test ordered: .... Test result: ....

....

....

....

Weight: .... Blood pressure: ....

Temperature: .... Heart rate: ....

Prescribed treatment:

Prescribed medications, vitamins, supplements:

Name: Dosage:

Frequency: Duration:

With meal and/or water?

Possible side effects:

NOTES

OFFICE VISIT

Date: .... Doctor: ....

Phone: .... Address: ....

....

Reason for visit: ....

....

....

....

....

Doctor's diagnosis/feedback: ....

....

....

....

....

....

Test ordered: .... Test result: ....

....

....

....

....

....

Weight: .... Blood pressure: ....

Temperature: .... Heart rate: ....

Prescribed treatment:

Prescribed medications, vitamins, supplements:

Name: Dosage:

Frequency: Duration:

With meal and/or water?

Possible side effects:

NOTES

NOTES

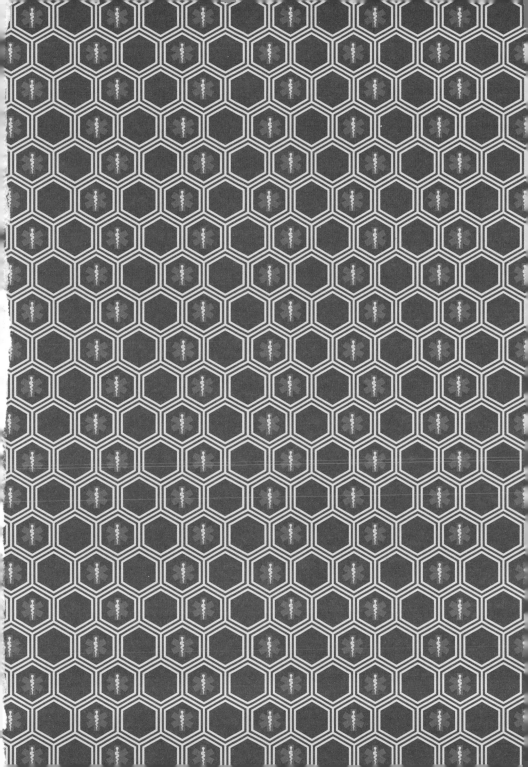

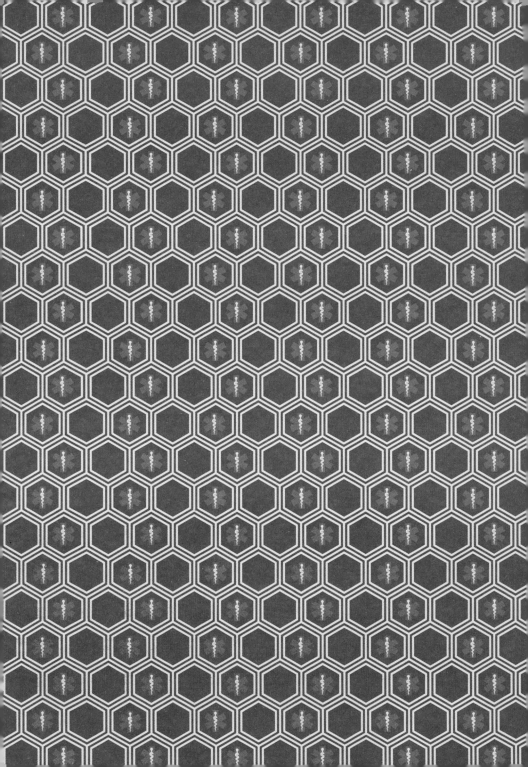